LOW PROTEIN DIET FOR KIDNEY DISEASE

Dr. Amy Olander

Copyright © 2024 by Dr. Amy Olander

Disclaimer

Every effort has been made to ensure that the recipes, cooking instructions, and nutritional information in this cookbook are accurate and reliable. However, cooking results may vary, and Dr. Amy is not responsible for any adverse effects or consequences that may result from the use of the information contained in this cookbook.

Dr. Amy and the publishers of this cookbook disclaim any liability or responsibility for any loss or damage incurred as a consequence of the recipes, cooking techniques, or dietary information provided in this cookbook. It is the reader's responsibility to exercise good judgment and ensure food safety when following these recipes.

Acknowledgment

Images in the cookbook by FREEPIK

TABLE OF CONTENT

Introduction... 5

    Understanding Kidney Health................................... 6

    Embarking on a Low Protein Culinary Journey...................... 7

RECIPES.. 9

    Vegetable Stir-Fry with Tofu..................................... 9

    Quinoa Salad with Roasted Vegetables............................. 10

    Lentil and Vegetable Soup.......................................11

    Baked Salmon with Lemon and Herbs............................ 12

    Eggplant and Zucchini Lasagna 13

    Chicken and Vegetable Skewers 14

    Spinach and Mushroom Omelette 15

    Cucumber and Tomato Salad 16

    Shrimp Stir-Fry with Broccoli.................................... 17

    Sweet Potato and Black Bean Tacos 18

    Grilled Turkey Burgers.. 19

    Cauliflower Fried Rice 20

    Roasted Cod with Asparagus..................................... 21

    Avocado and Chickpea Salad 22

    Turkey and Vegetable Meatballs 23

    Caprese Salad with Balsamic Glaze............................... 24

    Lemon Herb Baked Chicken 25

    Zucchini Noodles with Pesto..................................... 26

    Baked Tilapia with Dill 26

    Chickpea and Spinach Curry..................................... 27

    Turkey and Quinoa Stuffed Peppers.............................. 28

    Broccoli and Cheddar Frittata 30

Grilled Portobello Mushrooms 31

Lemon Garlic Shrimp Skewers 32

Roasted Brussels Sprouts with Cranberries 33

Conclusion 35

Introduction

Welcome to Low Protein Recipes for Kidney Disease. In this carefully curated collection, we invite you to embark on a flavorful exploration of wholesome, kidney-friendly cuisine designed to support and enhance your renal health.

Understanding the pivotal role nutrition plays in managing kidney disease is the cornerstone of our culinary adventure. Within these pages, we delve into the intricacies of kidney health, offering insights into the impact of a low protein diet on well-being. It's not merely about restrictions but a celebration of crafting delicious meals that nourish both body and soul.

Embarking on a Low Protein Culinary Journey, our introductory section, serves as a compass for readers navigating the realm of kidney-friendly living. We illuminate the significance of a low protein diet, providing a roadmap to not only meet dietary restrictions but to relish the delightful fusion of flavors in every dish.

As you flip through these pages, you'll catch a tantalizing glimpse of the culinary wonders awaiting you. From Vegetable Stir-Fry with Tofu to Quinoa Salad with Roasted Vegetables, our recipes showcase the harmonious blend of nutrition and taste. We aim to transform the perception of a low protein diet from a medical necessity into a gastronomic adventure, where every meal is a nourishing ode to well-being.

Join us in this culinary compassion for kidneys, where we believe that every bite contributes to your journey of health and vitality. Let's make the kitchen a space of healing, one delicious recipe at a time.

Kidneys play a pivotal role in maintaining the body's overall health and balance. These bean-shaped organs filter waste products and excess fluids from the bloodstream, regulate blood pressure, and produce hormones that control red blood cell production and calcium metabolism.

For individuals managing kidney disease, understanding the intricate workings of these vital organs is paramount. Kidney disease can stem from various factors, including diabetes, high blood pressure, genetic predispositions, and certain medications. Over time, impaired kidney function can lead to a buildup of toxins and fluid retention, posing significant health risks if left unmanaged.

Adopting a low protein diet is one of the cornerstones of kidney disease management. Protein breakdown produces waste products, such as urea and creatinine, which healthy kidneys filter out of the bloodstream. However, in individuals with compromised kidney function, excessive protein intake can strain the kidneys and exacerbate the progression of kidney disease.

A low protein diet aims to reduce the burden on the kidneys by limiting the amount of protein consumed while ensuring adequate nutrition and energy intake. By moderating protein intake, individuals can help slow the decline of kidney function and alleviate symptoms associated with kidney disease.

In addition to managing protein intake, other dietary considerations include monitoring sodium, potassium, and phosphorus levels. These electrolytes can accumulate in the bloodstream when kidney function is compromised, leading to fluid imbalances and electrolyte disturbances. Therefore, a balanced approach to nutrition is essential for supporting kidney health and overall well-being.

Embarking on a Low Protein Culinary Journey

Embarking on a low protein culinary journey is more than a dietary adjustment; it's a commitment to transforming the way we view food, flavors, and nourishment. This section serves as your compass in navigating the realm of kidney-friendly living, where we unravel the essential components of this culinary expedition.

1. Understanding the Significance: Embrace the profound impact a low protein diet can have on managing kidney disease. Recognize the role of dietary choices in alleviating strain on the kidneys and supporting overall renal health. This journey begins with awareness — understanding the why behind the dietary adjustments.

2. Celebrating Flavorful Fusion: Banish the misconception that a low protein diet equates to bland and uninspiring meals. Instead, anticipate a symphony of flavors as diverse ingredients come together in delightful combinations. Our recipes showcase the art of balancing taste and nutrition, proving that low protein doesn't mean compromising on culinary pleasure.

3. Navigating Dietary Choices: Navigate the landscape of dietary options with confidence. Learn to make informed decisions about protein sources, exploring alternatives that are gentle on the kidneys yet rich in essential nutrients. This journey involves not only what to include but also understanding the delicate balance of other vital nutrients, such as sodium, potassium, and phosphorus.

4. A Mindful Approach to Cooking: Transition to a mindful approach in the kitchen, where each ingredient is chosen purposefully and each preparation is a conscious step toward well-being. Discover the joy of experimenting with herbs, spices, and cooking techniques that enhance flavors without compromising renal health. This is a culinary adventure that emphasizes quality, variety, and creativity.

5. Transforming Perspectives: Shift your perspective from restriction to empowerment. This culinary journey is an opportunity to take control of your health through the joy of cooking and savoring nourishing meals. It's a celebration of the possibilities that unfold when we embrace a low protein diet not as a limitation, but as a foundation for building a healthier, more vibrant life.

RECIPES

Vegetable Stir-Fry with Tofu

Servings: 4
Prep Time: 15 minutes
Cooking Time: 15 minutes

Ingredients:

- 1 block firm tofu, cubed
- 2 cups broccoli florets
- 1 red bell pepper, sliced
- 1 yellow bell pepper, sliced
- 1 carrot, julienned
- 1 cup snap peas, ends trimmed
- 3 cloves garlic, minced
- 2 tablespoons soy sauce
- 1 tablespoon sesame oil
- 1 tablespoon olive oil
- 1 teaspoon ginger, grated
- 2 green onions, sliced
- Sesame seeds for garnish

Instructions:

1. Press tofu to remove excess water, then cube it.

2. Warm up the olive oil in a wok or big frying pan on medium-high heat.

3. Add tofu cubes and stir-fry until golden brown. Take the tofu out of the pan and set aside.

4. In the same pan, add sesame oil, garlic, and ginger. Sauté until fragrant.

5. Add broccoli, bell peppers, carrot, and snap peas. Stir-fry until vegetables are crisp-tender.

6. Return tofu to the pan, add soy sauce, and toss to combine.

7. Garnish with green onions and sesame seeds. Serve over rice or noodles.

Quinoa Salad with Roasted Vegetables

Servings: 6
Prep Time: 20 minutes
Cooking Time: 25 minutes

Ingredients:

- ➢ 1 cup quinoa, rinsed
- ➢ 2 cups cherry tomatoes, halved
- ➢ 1 zucchini, diced
- ➢ 1 red onion, sliced
- ➢ 1 red bell pepper, diced
- ➢ 3 tablespoons olive oil
- ➢ 2 tablespoons balsamic vinegar
- ➢ 1 teaspoon dried oregano
- ➢ Salt and pepper to taste
- ➢ Feta cheese for garnish (optional)
- ➢ Fresh basil for garnish

Instructions:

1. Preheat oven to 400°F (200°C).

2. Toss zucchini, red onion, and red bell pepper with 2 tablespoons of olive oil. Roast in the oven for 20-25 minutes or until vegetables are tender.

3. Cook quinoa according to package instructions.

4. In a large bowl, combine cooked quinoa, roasted vegetables, cherry tomatoes, oregano, balsamic vinegar, and remaining olive oil. Season with salt and pepper.

5. Garnish with crumbled feta cheese and fresh basil. Serve chilled.

Lentil and Vegetable Soup

Servings: 8
Prep Time: 15 minutes
Cooking Time: 40 minutes

Ingredients:

- ➢ 1 cup dried lentils, rinsed
- ➢ 1 onion, chopped
- ➢ 2 carrots, diced
- ➢ 2 celery stalks, chopped
- ➢ 3 cloves garlic, minced
- ➢ 1 can (14 oz) diced tomatoes
- ➢ 6 cups vegetable broth
- ➢ 1 teaspoon cumin
- ➢ 1 teaspoon paprika
- ➢ 1 bay leaf
- ➢ Salt and pepper to taste
- ➢ Fresh parsley for garnish

Instructions:

1. In a big pot, cook onions, carrots, and celery until they become soft.

2. Add garlic, cumin, and paprika. Stir for a minute until fragrant.

3. Pour in vegetable broth, lentils, diced tomatoes, and add a bay leaf. Bring to a boil, then reduce heat and simmer for 30-35 minutes or until lentils are tender.

4. Sprinkle with just the right amount of salt and pepper to suit your taste.

5. Garnish with fresh parsley before serving.

Baked Salmon with Lemon and Herbs

Servings: 4
Prep Time: 10 minutes
Cooking Time: 20 minutes

Ingredients:

- ➢ 4 salmon fillets
- ➢ 2 tablespoons olive oil
- ➢ 2 cloves garlic, minced
- ➢ 1 teaspoon dried thyme
- ➢ 1 teaspoon dried rosemary
- ➢ Zest of 1 lemon
- ➢ Juice of 1 lemon
- ➢ Salt and pepper to taste
- ➢ Fresh parsley for garnish

Instructions:

1. Preheat oven to 375°F (190°C).

2. Lay the salmon fillets on a baking sheet covered with parchment paper.

3. In a small bowl, mix olive oil, garlic, thyme, rosemary, lemon zest, and lemon juice.

4. Brush the mixture over the salmon fillets. Season with salt and pepper.

5. Bake for 18-20 minutes or until the salmon flakes easily with a fork.

6. Garnish with fresh parsley before serving.

Eggplant and Zucchini Lasagna

Servings: 6
Prep Time: 30 minutes
Cooking Time: 45 minutes

Ingredients:

- ➢ 1 large eggplant, thinly sliced
- ➢ 2 zucchinis, thinly sliced
- ➢ 1 onion, chopped
- ➢ 3 cloves garlic, minced
- ➢ 1 can (14 oz) crushed tomatoes
- ➢ 1 teaspoon dried oregano
- ➢ 1 teaspoon dried basil
- ➢ Salt and pepper to taste
- ➢ 2 cups ricotta cheese
- ➢ 1 cup shredded mozzarella cheese
- ➢ 1/2 cup grated Parmesan cheese
- ➢ Fresh basil for garnish

Instructions:

1. Preheat oven to 375°F (190°C).

2. In a skillet, sauté onions and garlic until softened. Add crushed tomatoes, oregano, basil, salt, and pepper and allow to Simmer for 10 minutes.

3. In a separate pan, grill eggplant and zucchini slices until lightly browned.

4. In a baking dish, layer grilled eggplant and zucchini, ricotta cheese, tomato sauce, and mozzarella. Repeat until ingredients are used, finishing with a layer of mozzarella and Parmesan cheese.

5. Bake for 35-40 minutes or until bubbly and golden.

6. Let it cool for 10 minutes, garnish with fresh basil, and serve.

Chicken and Vegetable Skewers

Servings: 4

Prep Time: 20 minutes

Cooking Time: 15 minutes

Ingredients:

- 1 lb boneless, skinless chicken breasts, cut into chunks
- Bell peppers (E.g. red, yellow, and green), cut into chunks
- Red onion, cut into chunks
- Cherry tomatoes
- Olive oil
- Lemon juice
- Garlic powder, salt, and pepper to taste

Instructions:

1. Preheat the grill or grill pan.

2. In a bowl, combine chicken chunks, bell peppers, red onion, and cherry tomatoes.

3. In a separate bowl, whisk together olive oil, lemon juice, garlic powder, salt, and pepper to make the marinade.

4. Thread the marinated chicken and vegetables onto skewers.

5. Grill skewers for about 15 minutes, turning occasionally, until chicken is cooked through.

6. Serve hot, optionally with a side of rice or a light salad.

Spinach and Mushroom Omelette

Servings: 2

Prep Time: 10 minutes

Cooking Time: 10 minutes

Ingredients:

- ➢ 4 large eggs
- ➢ 1 cup fresh spinach, chopped
- ➢ 1/2 cup mushrooms, sliced
- ➢ 1/4 cup feta cheese, crumbled
- ➢ Salt and pepper to taste
- ➢ Olive oil or cooking spray

Instructions:

1. In a bowl, whisk the eggs and season with salt and pepper.

2. Heat olive oil or cooking spray in a non-stick skillet over medium heat.

3. Add mushrooms to the skillet and sauté until they release moisture.

4. Toss in some chopped spinach into the pan and let it cook until it wilts.

5. Pour the whisked eggs over the vegetables, tilting the pan to spread them evenly.

6. Sprinkle crumbled feta cheese on top.

7. Once the edges set, carefully flip the omelette and cook until fully set.

8. Fold the omelette in half and serve hot.

Cucumber and Tomato Salad

Servings: 4

Prep Time: 15 minutes

Ingredients:

- ➢ 2 cucumbers, thinly sliced
- ➢ 2 cups cherry tomatoes, halved
- ➢ Red onion, thinly sliced
- ➢ 1/4 cup fresh basil, chopped
- ➢ Feta cheese, crumbled
- ➢ Olive oil, balsamic vinegar, salt, and pepper for taste

Instructions:

1. In a large bowl, combine sliced cucumbers, cherry tomatoes, red onion, and chopped basil.

2. In a small bowl, whisk together olive oil, balsamic vinegar, salt, and pepper to make the dressing.

3. Pour the dressing evenly onto the salad and give it a gentle toss to mix everything together.

4. Top with crumbled feta cheese before serving.

5. Serve chilled.

Shrimp Stir-Fry with Broccoli

Servings: 3

Prep Time: 15 minutes

Cooking Time: 10 minutes

Ingredients:

- 1 lb shrimp, peeled and deveined
- Broccoli florets
- Bell peppers, thinly sliced
- Soy sauce
- Garlic, minced
- Ginger, grated
- Sesame oil
- Red pepper flakes (optional)

Instructions:

1. In a wok or a big frying pan, warm up the sesame oil on medium-high heat.

2. Add shrimp and stir-fry until pink and opaque. Remove shrimp from the pan.

3. In the same pan, stir-fry broccoli and bell peppers until crisp-tender.

4. Add minced garlic and grated ginger to the vegetables; sauté for 1-2 minutes.

5. Return the cooked shrimp to the pan.

6. Pour soy sauce over the mixture and toss to combine.

7. If desired, sprinkle red pepper flakes for added heat.

8. Serve over rice or noodles.

Sweet Potato and Black Bean Tacos

Servings: 4

Prep Time: 20 minutes

Cooking Time: 25 minutes

Ingredients:

- ➢ 2 sweet potatoes, peeled and diced
- ➢ 1 can black beans, drained and rinsed
- ➢ Corn tortillas
- ➢ Avocado, sliced
- ➢ Lime wedges
- ➢ Cilantro, chopped
- ➢ Taco seasoning, cumin, and paprika
- ➢ Olive oil

Instructions:

1. Preheat the oven to 400°F (200°C).

2. Toss diced sweet potatoes in olive oil and season with taco seasoning, cumin, and paprika.

3. Roast sweet potatoes in the oven until tender, about 20-25 minutes.

4. In a skillet, warm black beans over medium heat.

5. Heat corn tortillas in a dry skillet or microwave.

6. Assemble tacos with roasted sweet potatoes, black beans, sliced avocado, and cilantro.

7. Serve with lime wedges on the side.

Grilled Turkey Burgers

Servings: 4

Prep Time: 15 minutes

Cooking Time: 15 minutes

Ingredients:

- ➤ 1 pound ground turkey
- ➤ 1/4 cup breadcrumbs
- ➤ 1 egg, beaten
- ➤ 1/4 cup finely chopped red onion
- ➤ 2 cloves garlic, minced
- ➤ 1 teaspoon dried oregano
- ➤ Salt and pepper to taste
- ➤ 4 whole-grain burger buns
- ➤ Lettuce, tomato, and other desired toppings

Instructions:

1. Preheat the grill to medium-high heat.

2. In a mixing bowl, combine ground turkey, breadcrumbs, beaten egg, red onion, minced garlic, oregano, salt, and pepper. Mix until well combined.

3. Separate the mix into four even parts and form them into patties for your burgers.

4. Place the patties on the preheated grill and cook for about 6-7 minutes per side or until fully cooked.

5. Toast the burger buns on the grill for 1-2 minutes.

6. Assemble the burgers by placing the turkey patties on the buns and adding your favorite toppings.

Cauliflower Fried Rice

Servings: 4

Prep Time: 10 minutes

Cooking Time: 15 minutes

Ingredients:

- ➢ 1 medium cauliflower, grated
- ➢ 2 tablespoons vegetable oil
- ➢ 1 cup diced carrots
- ➢ 1 cup frozen peas
- ➢ 2 cloves garlic, minced
- ➢ 2 eggs, beaten
- ➢ 3 tablespoons soy sauce
- ➢ 1 teaspoon sesame oil
- ➢ Green onions for garnish

Instructions:

1. Warm up some vegetable oil in a big pan or wok on medium heat.

2. Add finely chopped garlic and cook for about 1 minute until it releases its aromatic fragrance.

3. Add diced carrots and cook for 3-4 minutes until slightly softened.

4. Push the vegetables to one side of the pan and pour the beaten eggs into the other side. Scramble the eggs until cooked through.

5. Add grated cauliflower and frozen peas to the pan. Stir everything together.

6. Pour soy sauce and sesame oil over the mixture, stirring well to combine.

7. Cook for an additional 5-7 minutes, or until the cauliflower is tender.

8. Garnish with chopped green onions before serving.

Roasted Cod with Asparagus

Servings: 2

Prep Time: 10 minutes

Cooking Time: 15 minutes

Ingredients:

- 2 cod fillets
- 1 bunch asparagus, trimmed
- 2 tablespoons olive oil
- 1 lemon, sliced
- 2 cloves garlic, minced
- Salt and pepper to taste
- Fresh parsley for garnish

Instructions:

1. Preheat the oven to 400°F (200°C).

2. Place the cod fillets and trimmed asparagus on a baking sheet.

3. Drizzle olive oil over the fish and vegetables. Sprinkle minced garlic, salt, and pepper.

4. Arrange lemon slices on top.

5. Bake in the oven, already heated up, for about 12-15 minutes or until the cod is fully cooked and easily flakes apart.

6. Garnish with fresh parsley before serving.

Avocado and Chickpea Salad

Servings: 4

Prep Time: 10 minutes

Ingredients:

- ➤ 2 ripe avocados, diced
- ➤ 1 can (15 oz) chickpeas (drained and rinsed)
- ➤ 1 cup cherry tomatoes, halved
- ➤ 1/4 cup red onion, finely chopped
- ➤ 2 tablespoons fresh cilantro, chopped
- ➤ 1 tablespoon olive oil
- ➤ 1 tablespoon lemon juice
- ➤ Salt and pepper to taste

Instructions:

1. In a large bowl, combine diced avocados, chickpeas, cherry tomatoes, red onion, and cilantro.

2. In a little bowl, mix up some olive oil, lemon juice, along with a pinch of salt and pepper.

3. Drizzle the dressing over the salad and give it a gentle toss to mix everything together.

4. You can enjoy it right away or keep it in the fridge until you're ready to dig in.

Turkey and Vegetable Meatballs

Servings: 6

Prep Time: 20 minutes

Cooking Time: 20 minutes

Ingredients:

- ➤ 1 pound ground turkey
- ➤ 1/2 cup breadcrumbs
- ➤ 1/4 cup grated Parmesan cheese
- ➤ 1/4 cup finely chopped onion
- ➤ 1/4 cup finely chopped bell pepper
- ➤ 1 clove garlic, minced
- ➤ 1 teaspoon dried oregano
- ➤ Salt and pepper to taste
- ➤ 1 egg, beaten
- ➤ Marinara sauce for serving

Instructions:

1. Preheat the oven to 375°F (190°C).

2. In a large bowl, combine ground turkey, breadcrumbs, Parmesan cheese, chopped onion, chopped bell pepper, minced garlic, oregano, salt, and pepper.

3. Add the beaten egg to the mixture and mix until well combined.

4. Shape the mixture into meatballs and place them on a baking sheet.

5. Bake in the preheated oven for 20 minutes or until the meatballs are cooked through and browned on the outside.

6. Serve with your favorite marinara sauce.

Caprese Salad with Balsamic Glaze

Servings: 4

Prep Time: 10 minutes

Cooking Time: 0 minutes

Ingredients:

- ➢ 4 large ripe tomatoes, sliced
- ➢ 1 pound fresh mozzarella cheese, sliced
- ➢ Fresh basil leaves
- ➢ 1/4 cup extra-virgin olive oil
- ➢ Salt and pepper to taste
- ➢ Balsamic glaze for drizzling

Instructions:

1. Arrange tomato and mozzarella slices alternately on a serving platter.

2. Tuck fresh basil leaves between the tomato and mozzarella slices.

3. Drizzle extra-virgin olive oil over the salad.

4. Add salt and pepper according to your preference.

5. Right before you serve, pour a good amount of balsamic glaze over the dish.

6. Serve it up right away and savor the explosion of delicious flavors.

Lemon Herb Baked Chicken

Servings: 4

Prep Time: 15 minutes

Cooking Time: 30 minutes

Ingredients:

- ➤ 4 boneless, skinless chicken breasts
- ➤ 2 lemons, juiced and zested
- ➤ 3 tablespoons olive oil
- ➤ 2 cloves garlic, minced
- ➤ 1 teaspoon dried oregano
- ➤ 1 teaspoon dried thyme
- ➤ Salt and pepper to taste
- ➤ Lemon slices for garnish

Instructions:

1. Preheat the oven to 400°F (200°C).

2. In a bowl, whisk together lemon juice, lemon zest, olive oil, minced garlic, oregano, thyme, salt, and pepper.

3. Place chicken breasts in a baking dish and pour the lemon herb mixture over them, ensuring even coating.

4. Bake for about 25-30 minutes or until chicken reaches an internal temperature of 165°F (74°C).

5. Garnish with lemon slices and serve with your favorite sides.

Servings: 3-4

Prep Time: 15 minutes

Cooking Time: 5 minutes

Ingredients:

- ➤ 4 medium zucchinis, spiralized into noodles
- ➤ 1 cup fresh basil leaves
- ➤ 1/2 cup grated Parmesan cheese
- ➤ 1/3 cup pine nuts
- ➤ 2 cloves garlic
- ➤ 1/2 cup extra-virgin olive oil
- ➤ Salt and pepper to taste
- ➤ Cherry tomatoes for garnish

Instructions:

1. In a food processor, combine basil, Parmesan, pine nuts, and garlic. Pulse until finely chopped.

2. With the processor running, slowly pour in the olive oil until the pesto reaches your desired consistency.

3. Season with salt and pepper.

4. In a pan over medium heat, sauté zucchini noodles for 3-5 minutes or until just tender.

5. Toss the zucchini noodles with the prepared pesto.

6. Garnish with cherry tomatoes and serve immediately.

Baked Tilapia with Dill

Servings: 2

Prep Time: 10 minutes

Cooking Time: 15 minutes

Ingredients:

- 2 tilapia fillets
- 2 tablespoons olive oil
- 2 tablespoons lemon juice
- 2 cloves garlic, minced
- 1 teaspoon dried dill
- Salt and pepper to taste
- Lemon wedges for serving

Instructions:

1. Preheat the oven to 400°F (200°C).

2. Place tilapia fillets in a baking dish.

3. In a small bowl, whisk together olive oil, lemon juice, minced garlic, dried dill, salt, and pepper.

4. Pour the mixture over the tilapia, ensuring even coating.

5. Bake the fish in the oven for 12-15 minutes, or just until it easily separates into flakes when prodded with a fork.

6. Serve with lemon wedges and enjoy this light and flavorful dish.

Chickpea and Spinach Curry

Servings: 4

Prep Time: 15 minutes

Cooking Time: 20 minutes

Ingredients:

- 1 can (15 oz) chickpeas, (drained and rinsed)
- 1 onion, finely chopped
- 2 cloves garlic, minced
- 1 tablespoon ginger, grated
- 1 can (14 oz) diced tomatoes
- 1 can (14 oz) coconut milk
- 2 teaspoons curry powder
- 1 teaspoon ground cumin
- 1 teaspoon ground coriander
- 1/2 teaspoon turmeric
- Salt and pepper to taste
- 4 cups fresh spinach leaves

Instructions:

1. In a large pan, sauté chopped onion until translucent.

2. Add minced garlic and grated ginger, cooking for an additional 2 minutes.

3. Stir in curry powder, cumin, coriander, and turmeric.

4. Add chickpeas, diced tomatoes, and coconut milk. Season with salt and pepper.

5. Simmer for 15-20 minutes, allowing flavors to meld and the curry to thicken.

6. Just before serving, stir in fresh spinach until wilted.

7. Serve over rice or with your preferred side.

Turkey and Quinoa Stuffed Peppers

Servings: 4

Prep Time: 20 minutes

Cooking Time: 40 minutes

Ingredients:

- 4 large bell peppers, halved and seeds removed
- 1 lb ground turkey
- 1 cup cooked quinoa
- 1 cup diced tomatoes
- 1/2 cup black beans, drained and rinsed
- 1/2 cup corn kernels
- 1/2 cup diced red onion
- 1 teaspoon cumin
- 1 teaspoon chili powder
- Salt and pepper to taste
- 1 cup shredded cheese (optional, for topping)

Instructions:

1. Preheat the oven to 375°F (190°C).

2. In a skillet over medium heat, cook the ground turkey until browned. Drain excess fat.

3. In a large bowl, combine cooked turkey, quinoa, diced tomatoes, black beans, corn, red onion, cumin, chili powder, salt, and pepper.

4. Fill each half of the bell pepper with the mixture of turkey and quinoa.

5. Place stuffed peppers in a baking dish and cover with aluminum foil.

6. Bake for 30 minutes, then remove the foil, sprinkle shredded cheese on top if desired, and bake for an

additional 10 minutes or until the cheese is melted and bubbly.

7. Serve hot and enjoy your Turkey and Quinoa Stuffed Peppers!

Broccoli and Cheddar Frittata

Servings: 6

Prep Time: 15 minutes

Cooking Time: 25 minutes

Ingredients:

- 8 large eggs
- 1 cup broccoli florets, steamed and chopped
- 1 cup shredded cheddar cheese
- 1/2 cup diced red bell pepper
- 1/4 cup diced onion
- Salt and pepper to taste
- 2 tablespoons olive oil

Instructions:

1. Preheat the oven to 375°F (190°C).

2. In a bowl, whisk together eggs, salt, and pepper.

3. Heat olive oil in an oven-safe skillet over medium heat. Saute onions and red bell pepper until softened.

4. Add steamed broccoli to the skillet and spread the vegetables evenly.

5. Pour the whisked eggs over the vegetables and let it cook for 2 minutes without stirring.

6. Sprinkle shredded cheddar cheese on top.

7. Transfer the skillet to the preheated oven and bake for 20-25 minutes or until the frittata is set in the middle.

8. Slice into wedges and serve your Broccoli and Cheddar Frittata warm.

Grilled Portobello Mushrooms

Servings: 2

Prep Time: 10 minutes

Cooking Time: 10 minutes

Ingredients:

➢ 2 large portobello mushrooms
➢ 2 tablespoons balsamic vinegar
➢ 2 tablespoons olive oil
➢ 2 cloves garlic, minced
➢ Salt and pepper to taste
➢ Fresh parsley for garnish (optional)

Instructions:

1. Preheat the grill to medium-high heat.

2. Wash the portobello mushrooms and take out the stems.

3. In a small bowl, whisk together balsamic vinegar, olive oil, minced garlic, salt, and pepper.

4. Brush the mushroom caps with the balsamic mixture.

5. Grill the mushrooms for 5 minutes on each side, or until tender.

6. Garnish with fresh parsley if desired.

7. Serve your Grilled Portobello Mushrooms as a flavorful side dish or on a salad.

Lemon Garlic Shrimp Skewers

Servings: 4

Prep Time: 15 minutes

Cooking Time: 6 minutes

Ingredients:

- 1 lb large shrimp, peeled and deveined
- 3 cloves garlic, minced
- Zest of 1 lemon
- Juice of 1 lemon
- 2 tablespoons olive oil
- 1 teaspoon dried oregano
- Salt and pepper to taste
- Wooden skewers, soaked in water for 30 minutes

Instructions:

1. Heat the grill or grill pan over medium-high heat.

2. In a bowl, combine minced garlic, lemon zest, lemon juice, olive oil, oregano, salt, and pepper.

3. Thread shrimp onto the soaked skewers.

4. Brush the shrimp skewers with the lemon-garlic marinade.

5. Grill the shrimp for 2 to 3 minutes on each side, or until they turn opaque and are thoroughly cooked.

6. Serve your Lemon Garlic Shrimp Skewers with a squeeze of fresh lemon juice.

Roasted Brussels Sprouts with Cranberries

Servings: 4

Prep Time: 10 minutes

Cooking Time: 25 minutes

Ingredients:

- 1 lb Brussels sprouts, trimmed and halved
- 1/2 cup dried cranberries
- 2 tablespoons olive oil
- 2 tablespoons balsamic vinegar
- Salt and pepper to taste
- 1/4 cup chopped pecans (for garnish)

Instructions:

1. Preheat the oven to 400°F (200°C).

2. In a large bowl, toss Brussels sprouts and dried cranberries with olive oil, balsamic vinegar, salt, and pepper.

3. Spread the blend evenly over a baking sheet.

4. Roast for 20-25 minutes or until Brussels sprouts are golden brown and tender, stirring halfway through.

5. Optional: Sprinkle chopped pecans over the roasted Brussels sprouts for added crunch.

6. Serve your Roasted Brussels Sprouts with Cranberries as a delightful side dish.

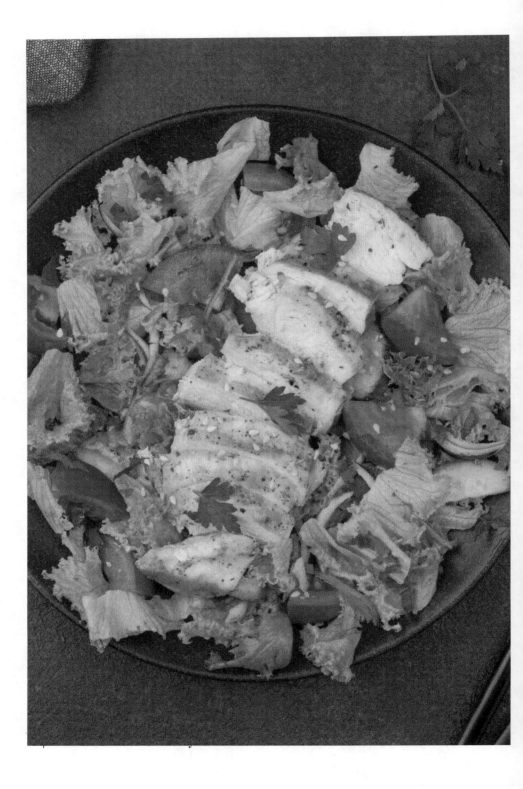

Conclusion

As we bid farewell to this culinary journey through **Low Protein Recipes for Kidney Disease**, we hope this collection of recipes has not just graced your kitchen but has become a companion in your pursuit of kidney health and overall well-being.

In the pages preceding this conclusion, we ventured into the intricacies of kidney health, discovering the profound impact of a low protein diet. We embarked on a journey that celebrated the fusion of flavors and proved that nourishing meals can be both delicious and mindful. Together, we navigated the culinary landscape, making informed choices to support kidney health while relishing the art of cooking.

Our recipes, from the Turkey and Quinoa Stuffed Peppers to the Grilled Portobello Mushrooms, were crafted with care and consideration. Each dish carries not just the essence of ingredients but also the intention to make your kitchen a space of healing. We aimed to transform the perception of a low protein diet from a medical necessity into a flavorful adventure where every bite contributes to your journey of health and vitality.

As you continue your path towards kidney wellness, we encourage you to savor the joy of preparing and sharing these meals with loved ones. Let each recipe be a reminder that a low protein diet isn't a restriction but an opportunity to explore the vast palette of culinary possibilities.

Thank you for inviting us into your kitchen and entrusting us with a small part of your health journey. May these recipes continue to nourish your body and delight your taste buds, making each meal a celebration of life, health, and the joy found in every flavorful bite.

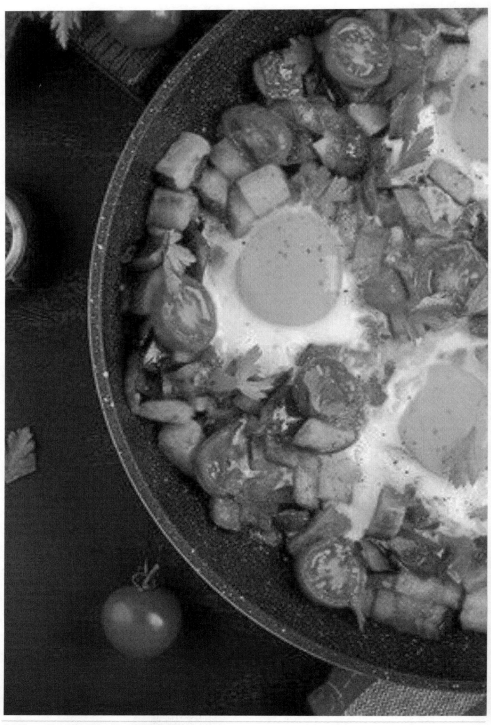

Made in United States
Troutdale, OR
07/17/2024

21272924R00022